Rumination
About
the Fruit of the Spirit

Goodness

A funny thing happened
on the way
to quitting smoking

I got a life

By
April Heather

Author April Heather
Edited by Dar Streedbeck
Photo credit Brett Allen
Printed by CreateSpace
Available on Kindle
Made in the United States of America
ISBN-13: 978-1503250956
ISBN- 10-1503250954

Other titles and new releases by April Heather

Also available on Kindle and other devices

Rumination About the Fruit of the Spirit: Patience
Rumination About the Fruit of the Spirit: Kindness

Soon to be released 2014

Rumination About the Fruit of the Spirit: Faithfulness
Rumination About the Fruit of the Spirit: Gentleness
Rumination About the Fruit of the Spirit: Self-control

Rumination About the Fruit of the Spirit: Goodness

"But the fruit of the spirit is

love, joy, peace,

patience, kindness, goodness,

faithfulness, gentleness and self-control.

Against such things there is no law."

Galatians 5:22, 23 NIV

"Let us not become conceited, provoking and

envying each other."

Galatians 5:26 NIV

Prologue

My grandmother was the best Christian in the world. It's just too bad I didn't respect the fact that she was. Back when I was between the ages of twelve and fourteen, I was too busy being mad at my warm and loving grandma for being a teacher and acting like one. Especially since she was retired from the local school district and especially since we weren't in school. We were at her kitchen table, at my favorite place in the whole world, my grandparent's farm in southeastern South Dakota; and she was wrecking it by being a teacher. When it came to school, any type of school, there was no rest for that woman. She was always dragging my younger sisters and me off to Sunday School, Vacation Bible School, church and then she would assign us homework with study books in math and English that she chose from the magazine rack in the grocery store.

In this particular instance, she was making us memorize Bible verses every day. My way of thinking was that it was summer and I could get that kind of grief at home during the school year. Why couldn't she just be a grandma? Well, she was being a grandma. My grandma. I suppose she was struggling too, because if she was a teacher, then why wasn't I a better student? Even more annoying, the two younger girls were rattling off their memorized pieces so well. Boy, did I get mad at that. When it came to this "fruit of the spirit" verse, I was fed up with the process and had had enough; I let her know it. It was probably the only time I ever won an argument with her. I knew it, too. It caught me off guard and I was surprised there wasn't more pleasure in winning. Even though it was no fun and games, the pressure was off and with that came relief.

Cut to fifteen years later; I was married with two children and I recognized this Bible verse immediately while I was driving home and saw it on a banner hanging from a church. I remember it being up there longer than any other banner that has ever been posted in this town, and it was there for me to ponder every day as I drove by. Since I didn't have to memorize the thing, I could now see the wisdom in it. When I got home, I showed my kids its location in Galatians and then wrote it down in the back of their Bibles. We discussed it a little bit and every once in while we will make a reference to "use your virtues" or "use your fruits." I DID NOT make them memorize it.

Well, just about another ten years after that, I was nearly 40 and a funny thing happened on the way to quitting smoking. It was Christmas time and as usual, I was preparing myself to quit smoking and eventually fail again for the new year. Everywhere I looked I saw LOVE, JOY, and PEACE and I remember thinking, "Where is the rest of it?" You know...the rest of the verse, because Grandma placed such a huge importance on memorizing the whole thing, not just the first three words. Then I got to thinking that everybody is constantly on the search for happiness and yet all the promotion stops after love, joy, and peace. That is when it occurred to me that maybe you can't get to the love, joy, and peace unless you first enact the patience, kindness, goodness, faithfulness, gentleness, and self-control.

Invigorated by my new epiphany, I made the decision to spend the next day looking for any and all ways to extend patience. It was a passive day, spent watching and learning, more than it was about controlling and doing. That night, I had gained so much information that I decided to do it again the very next day. The third and fourth day, I took a break to be normal for a couple of days. I didn't want to hold myself accountable for not meeting new standards of behavior. That seemed exhausting. I was looking for love, joy, and peace. I was looking for freedom. I was looking for a way to stabilize my life so I could allow the process of withdrawal to happen when I quit smoking. During the third and fourth days, I tried to go about my day normally while weighing my new information against life's usual routine. A couple days later, I did the practice all over again, except I moved on to the virtue of kindness. I kept at it until I had made it through the remaining six fruits of the verse.

From the get-go I had mini-explosions of epiphany after epiphany. I decided to postpone my New Year's quit date and I kept on going with the next virtue. Most of this was about watching and learning; at this time I wasn't after any permanent changes to my attitude or routine. I got curious ... then tested it to see what would happen. I did do a round two with the intent to apply some changes and I found it didn't require an overhaul of my life. It mostly was the result of, "If you know better you do better" (Maya Angelou).

Talk about a slow learner! I had thought I was having trouble learning the verse sitting at the kitchen table with my grandma and look what I just admitted to you. Learning a lesson after what -- twenty-five years maybe? You know, I had never really wanted to re-live my childhood, nor do I want a do-over. But man, if I could have applied this to my twenties right before I became a parent ... that would have been ... Wow! ... to have learned how to handle stress instead of avoiding it. ... To have been seated comfortably inside my own character ... at rest in my parental resolve. It would have been career changing ... life changing! At least I think all these things, because I am feeling pretty good right now. Some of this good feeling could have come with age but still ... I could've and should've known then what I know now ... because I knew this verse back then. Now, the best I can do is pass my lessons on to others like me and to the next generation.

Maybe I oversimplify when I boil all the answers into one single Bible verse, because there is more to reducing stress and living a balanced lifestyle, but this verse sums it up pretty well. (Gal. 5:22, 23 NIV) "But the fruit of the spirit is love, joy, peace, patience, kindness, goodness, faithfulness, gentleness, and self-control. Against such things there is no law." Soon after it, verse 26 says, "Let us not become conceited, provoking, and envying each other." As I put each virtue into daily practice, I came to view the Fruits of the Spirit as the "do's" and most of the Ten Commandments as the "don'ts."

Just take a moment to think this over ... if you concentrate on these virtues, you don't have to worry about breaking the law because against such things there are no laws. In today's over-regulated world, there might be a few regulations to enforce the positive; but for the most part, our laws are a preventive maintenance tool to control the negative.

Now to be sure, I am not talking about crisis mode. I am talking about everyday living, and life darting from moment to moment. You know at some point in the next few hours that someone or something is going to clamor for your attention. The moment is yours to respond: are you going to choose a fruit to apply to the distraction, or are you going to get exasperated at the source?

In keeping with my epiphany that "you need to enact the rest of the verse to achieve the love, joy, and peace," I wrote my experiences with Patience in one book, Kindness in another book, and a book each for Goodness, Faithfulness, Gentleness, and Self-control. Six books in all. They don't have to be read in any particular order. For that reason this prologue accompanies all of them and you only need to read this once. In the next book, you can get started right away with Chapter One.

With that, we will pick the fruit of the day. Let's see ... which one did you choose ... ?

Goodness (paraphrased due to all the uses)

Good: adjective
1. to be desired or approved of
2. having the qualities required for a particular role, purpose or cause
3. possessing or displaying moral virtue or principles by showing kindness, obedience, respect, or relating to social class, with other uses considered to be humorous or patronizing
4. Giving pleasure that is enjoyable, pleasant, attractive, or satisfying
5. Thorough, as in a good cleaning, or a good look around. Or emphasis as in a good long hug
6. used in exclamation of extreme surprise or anger: good heavens! Good gravy!

Good: noun
1. that which is morally right, righteousness
2. of benefit or advantage to someone or something
3. (goods) merchandise or possessions

Good: adverb
1.   well: as in done good or my mother could never cook this good.

Goodness: noun
The quality of being good; in particular, virtues, moral excellence or the beneficial or nourishing element of food.
                                   -2010 New Oxford American Dictionary
                                                              3rd edition

Thesaurus

Prologue

goodness: noun
1. (ex: She must have seen some goodness in him) virtue, good, righteousness, morality, integrity, rectitude, honesty, truth, truthfulness, honor, probity, propriety, decency, respectability, nobility, worthiness, worth, merit, trustworthiness, blamelessness, purity.

2. (ex: The neighbor's goodness toward us) kindness, kindliness, tenderheartedness, humanity, mildness, benevolence, graciousness, tenderness, warmth, affection, love, goodwill, sympathy, compassion, care, concern, understanding, tolerance, generosity, charity, leniency, clemency, magnanimity.

3. (ex: slow cooking retains the food's goodness) nutritional value, nutrients.

-2008 Oxford American Writer's Thesaurus
2nd edition

Goodness

Chapter 1   Goodness

I was apprehensive about beginning my work on Goodness. I anticipated that I would have to come up with a bunch of "Random Acts of Kindness." After all, isn't being kind to others the definition of spreading Goodness?

But I had recently recovered from burn-out, and quite frankly, I didn't want to get swept up with grand gestures and return to doing for others until I overdid it. In my former scatter-brained world, to do one surprise — such as stopping on the way to the bank to buy donuts for the tellers, and get them through the drive-up drawer — although a good idea, can seem overwhelming, especially when squashed between errands.

I resisted the concept that I simply needed to put some practice into being generous of spirit, as if a toggle switch would flip me from being drawn out, tired, and disgruntled, to being loving, joyful, and peaceful. Ta-da! Just because I'm doing for others! Isn't that how life's lessons are presented to us? Isn't that how we interpret this information? I thought of skipping Goodness, but I was doing this fruity project because I figured there was something to learn from each virtue. I didn't want to cheat, then miss out on the benefit of the lesson.

I resisted working on Goodness because I believed being "good" and putting others before me had gotten me into trouble in the first place. How could I use it for correction, when it was the very mistake that had put me there? Several times I wondered, "Why couldn't I just do lots of little, almost insignificant acts that add up to a good day? Could small acts of just saying, 'Thank you' and 'You're welcome,' be enough?"

About this time, I had narrowed it down to two problem areas: not enough time and guilt. With time … If someone asked for my help while I was in the middle of something, I knew my stuff would get done whenever I got around to it, so I usually stopped to help. I believed that was being "good," because I had put others before me. Since I was recovering from burnout, I so desperately needed it to be **my** turn, but how could that happen while working on goodness? … unless someone actually gave me my turn and that wasn't happening. It seemed like I couldn't be good enough to receive that award.

The problem was, since there are only so many hours in the day, all I had time for were the crappier things that I wanted. Such as, laundry, scrubbing floors, balancing the checkbook. I was always going to the grocery store between ten and midnight, when instead I should've been in bed. Wow! I just said that the highlight of my day was scrubbing the floor and not something special. This was not my dream life! No wonder I was done with being nice.

Goodness

Enter guilt … Well, to simplify, I'm done wearing guilt.

I can say that because I am responsible and I'm not trying to avoid consequences.

These guilty charges are so subtle we take them as normal. Most nearly slip right by. Case in point, I noticed I began to wince at the term "giving back." It seems as though the term has been tossed around as a guilt trip for people having what they have, even if it's not much. As if they didn't work hard enough to earn it in the first place, now they need to work some more … after the fact. It's a jab to get good people to be "gooder." I had jumped on this "giving back" bandwagon at one point, until it was used in my general direction and I stopped to consider, "Don't I do enough? How much more am I supposed to **do**?"

Think about it. Who tracks who has given back and who hasn't? Who judges how much I took and sees if I gave enough back? There are people with unmet needs who give, so **what** are they giving **back**? If people give back out of a sense of misplaced guilt, they lose the lesson in knowing how to receive. But some people fear that others receive too much, as if someone must control the distribution (one of many reasons why I no longer worry about playing fair).

Performing "Random Acts of Kindness" and volunteering are important, but I think we get stuck in the learning phase, afraid that we'll forget the lesson … Or we think the things we give up freely and independently don't count, because we don't feel the pressure. As if it isn't demanding enough. Giving and sacrifice are supposed to be hard, right? Does it still count if "doing" is easy? What if giving 110% were easy? I am taking a moment to test whether **maybe**, if it's easy, it's possible I'm in the right place at the right time. If it is easy, maybe I am being myself — not trying to be someone else; perhaps if it's hard, maybe I shouldn't follow through.

My question for my practice day on Goodness was, how could I recognize all this, and still be a good person spreading Goodness?

Chapter 2   Accountability vs. Responsibility

Accountability and responsibility are practically interchangeable words. It seems you can almost always use responsibility in place of accountability, but you wouldn't always use accountability instead of responsibility. For example, you wouldn't say that someone grew up to be accountable; you'd say that person grew up to be responsible ... labeling someone accountable gives a slightly different image. To me the definitions become vastly different when I notice that I don't have a problem telling people to stop being accountable, but I have a **huge** problem with telling people to stop being responsible.

By the time I had come upon this fruity experiment, I was so disenfranchised from everything: I had trouble getting through a simple conversation. Come on! I'm blonde, blue eyed, a bit top heavy, I sprinkle powder blue and Barbie pink everywhere I go. Now I'm spouting Bible verses. What do you **think** I'm consistently challenged with?

I previously thought all I had to do was to be patient and work around this perception of the "dumb blonde" until we'd get back to the matter at hand. Then there was an inexplicable shift in my life when conversations deteriorated before they even began. So, I started there: What would happen if I shut up and let others do all the talking? I was amazed at the results. Some of my relationships changed and I found out who was toxic and who wasn't. That started a cascade of testing the opposite of my usual perspective.

What would happen if I didn't take the lead?
What would happen if I didn't accept accountability?
What if I wasn't involved in everything?
What if I didn't speak up?
… If I didn't work extra hours?
… If I didn't share?
… If I didn't do my part?
… If I didn't apologize?
What would happen if I didn't go above and beyond what was called for?
… If I only did the minimum?
… If I only did what I had the time and energy for?
What would happen if I quit worrying about others and I watched out for me?
What would happen if I did the things that I liked but nothing else? Without having to withstand all the b.s. of "earning" those things?

Resolving each of these questions took a lot of patience and self-control as I watched for the outcome. It was a struggle because not taking action invites fear of subsequent fallout, for which I'd be accountable. I was putting up a fight against the fear of being labeled one of "those" people … those lazy people who don't earn their keep.

Accountability vs. Responsibility

Through it all, I wondered what went wrong until it made my head spin. You know, I grew up a couple of decades ago and I still get into trouble. What is that? What challenges your perception of being an adult and says you're naughty? No matter where I was in life, or what job I had, or how old my kids were, I always felt the same pressure to invite accountability in the name of being responsible; not just for me but on behalf of other people, too. We circle around that pressure and feed off of each other.

Since when did accountability become a badge of honor? What IS that? What is it that makes you want to do, and do, and do, to upset the balance in the name of finding the balance? Can't you be responsible without being held accountable?

What is it in life that makes you feel guilty?
What is it that makes you feel so wrong?
Why is it you can never do enough? Then still more needs to be done.
Did you spend too much money?
Could you have allocated your time differently?
Did you miss that promotion at work?
Could you have done more, tried harder?
What is it that makes you feel like you aren't worthy to take your vacation or use your sick days?
Did you say the wrong thing in a conversation?
Do you need to go back and redo the conversation?
Did you eat healthy meals this week?
Could you have allocated more time to cook those meals?
Did you kill your houseplants?
Have you hugged your kid today?

Goodness

Did you skip dusting this week?

Do you live out of the clean laundry basket, because you never get the clothes put away?

Instead of accomplishing it all, did exercising replace vacuuming?

Are you habitually late?

Are you habitually late, and things still aren't done as they "should" be?

Then what is your excuse for being late? ... all the time?

Are you constantly being challenged right down to the lightest "tsk" in a conversation to the shortest "eh," when working with others?

Are you spinning "should've" and "could've" around, and you can't shut it off because you're in s-o-o-o much trouble?

Why are you going to be in trouble?

Who are you going to be in trouble with?

What is going to happen?

Is God going to reach down from the heavens and give you a spanking?

You are an adult now. You're not naughty, naughty, naughty! And, you weren't put on this earth to make others feel naughty, either.

I repeat ... Can't you be responsible without being held accountable?

Isn't that what adults do? Isn't that what being an adult IS? I need to tell you that easing up on the accountability is so much better than being worried sick while waiting for the great equalizer to stab me even harder with an unexpected bill, a busted water pipe, car troubles, or putting a loved one in the hospital. These aren't things to punish me for past sins or to negate any recent successes. These are new tests to be my best in reaching a solution.

What if we pretend everyone is responsible and let everyone be accountable for only **their** mistakes and leave it at that? When mistakes happen, what if we skip the accountability and move right into the recovery? Do you think that's unreliable and everyone will run amok? Think about it. You consider yourself responsible, so enact the Golden Rule … remember that is "Treat others how you want to be treated." Not, "Do unto others how you **think** they would treat you, and do it first, before they get a chance to do it to you."

Are you saying others should act like you aren't responsible even though you are? I'm telling you; if it's not your fault, butt out.

For one day, you should go without doling out accountability, avoid accepting it, and if you make a mistake, step up and fix it without apologizing. Don't explain away any mistakes with a long string of excuses. Don't go pointing out the mistakes you made. Don't point out and fix other people's mistakes. Just for one day, set aside your ego and see if you can find little nuances between being responsible and doing more than you need too. You should be able to do this without making yourself look bad **because** you are a responsible person.

Goodness

Chapter 3   Gratitude

As well as feeling accountable for everything, I felt that I wasn't allowed to whine, either. I thought that was unfair, since I had to listen to other people whine whenever they were victims of circumstance. When it was **my** turn to whine, I was told that I shouldn't feel bad, since there are people who don't have it as good ... usually noting there's always starving children in Africa, China, or India. Am I supposed to keep my mouth shut and never complain, never try to figure things out, because I should shut up and be grateful?

I loathed the statement, "Other people have it worse," so much, I quit saying it, myself. Even though its intent is to quit being negative and accentuate the positive, it just doesn't comfort people the way you expect positive thinking should. For this reason, gratitude is what always started my downward spiral.

I'll tell you, whenever I counted my blessings, I would end up feeling worse than when I started. I felt like I was being told I couldn't grow anymore. I was grateful for my family and I wanted to do more for them. Yet, if I'm to shut up and be grateful, does that mean, I'm not supposed to want for anything more? Then I'd start to compare things. "It's so unfair that other people get to pursue their goals and I don't! Lots of people can make more money in forty hours and one job than I do working sixty hours in three jobs."

I wanted to be home more. I wanted to use that time to be with family instead of cleaning house and getting mad that I had to clean … I could go on. That's why people were telling me to shut up, because others have it worse. Then my next downward spiral would start: "Well, other people can have success. I'm worthy and capable, so why doesn't it come my way?" I just want to do what I'm supposed to do as a human … to quit striving and start living.

My whining was from trying to get unstuck so I could find success. When people didn't want to listen, they would instead tell me to quit whining and be grateful. It was like telling me I don't matter; only those who have it worse than me matter. There will always be people who are worse off than me, so with that rationale, I will never matter … speaking of which, some would respond to my whining with, "Think that's bad?" and I would find myself in a competition for whose hardships were more relevant. What's more, when someone tells me to be grateful because others have it worse — I'm horrified that I should feel lucky due to someone else's hardships. Pick your spiral; each one has its own slippery slope.

Finally, I was able to separate myself from the spiral. I decided we are all individuals and I was going to find my uniqueness unrelated to anything or anyone else. Instead of waking up and acknowledging a list of blessings before my feet hit the floor, I woke up and asked, "What will God gift me with today?" This aroused my curiosity to get out of bed, to quit worrying about everyone else, and to find my new thing to be grateful for. Besides, whoever said that I was never grateful for the stuff I already had?

I got curious to find something new to be grateful for ... AND it worked. I tell you, the dread and limitations fell away and I received all of it, both material and immaterial. I received small amounts of money unexpectedly. I went on little trips even though I didn't think I could afford them. I was "doing lunch" when — now that I had the time, I didn't have the money. I witnessed the awe of jaw-dropping skylines. I disappeared into the beauty of a flower. I helped plot celebrations and kind gestures.

This became its own exercise separate from the Fruit of the Spirit exercise I had been working on. I dropped all expectations. I didn't coerce what I wanted to receive, so that I could see it materialize in a few days. I merely noticed what I received. I didn't turn anything away, I merely took it and said, "Thank you." I didn't have to keep it. I didn't have to like it. It didn't have to fit. I cognitively lined up all my gifts for which to be accounted. Some things weren't around to count as I had passed them on already. There was no deal breaker. I could enjoy it, pass it on, throw it away, or fix it. After only about two weeks of seeking out God's gifts for me, I was able to use the gratitude exercise for what it is and truly enjoy everything for which I'm grateful.

This exercise in being grateful was also a big lesson in learning how to receive, especially since I had wondered what in the heck I was giving back when I thought I never received anything. Maybe I had been turning some of it away. While I don't receive government assistance, nor get aid from any organization, I did notice that I received more then I realized. My landscaping is awesome because I started small, let it multiply, and added free divisions from my neighbors. A lot of free flowers. I received a kiln from someone who'd closed their ceramic business long ago and was tired of holding on to it forever. Out of all the people or organizations she could give it to, she gave it to me. With each of these gifts I was to shut up and say, "Thank you." Not protest nor profess my unworthiness, nor wonder why in the heck did I receive this out-dated jean jacket I didn't want. I used few words and just said, "Thank you."

Being thankful for immaterial things doesn't mean you should be ashamed of material ones. Gratefulness is not a one or the other deal. You know, those material things keep people working. They keep people fed. Those material things make other people thankful for having a roof over their head and the ability to provide for their family. Material things drive creativity and innovation. Why do we attach shame to this, then whine when all our production jobs go overseas?

Just because some people need to lay off buying into every fad, doesn't mean that everyone who shops is materialistic. Right now, the way I see it is, if I go around seeking my share of "everything," my life will get bumped off track and lose momentum. That doesn't mean I can't "want." In most cases, it means don't be distracted by what others have. Instead, I go after what I want and not with a feverish, no-holds-barred, competitive pitch.

Gratitude

Just don't be ruthless and vindictive, but live life as it comes and pay attention along the way. To do that takes Patience, Faith and Self-control and a reminder to be kind, good and gentle while you go after what you want.

Goodness

Chapter 4   I'm Not Naughty, Naughty, Naughty

I can't make people happy, but I sure can piss them off. I'm done getting caught up in another person's sentiment about the moment, at my expense.

I have wondered, how is it that I am expected to cow to someone else's temperament, meaning that I should fall in line, but when I try to command the same respect, I'm not taken seriously? How come what I put out there doesn't come back?

Take a minute to think about this threat, "You behave or I'll get mad," means, I just handed control of my emotions to you. I just offered to be your puppet since I gave you the choice to make me happy or make me mad. With this epiphany, my emotions aren't a part of the deal anymore. I want to protect my good day. To be clear, if you chose to get mad about something I did, the "I'm not naughty, naughty, naughty; I'm an adult," is a declaration I'd use for myself and not a statement I'd yell back at you.

How did we get here? I've heard, (but don't know who to credit) that this "naughty reaction" starts when we are children and don't want to see the scowl on a parent's face, while preferring the smile. From then on, we are caught in the dilemma that doing good is rewarded with good behavior from others and doing bad invites bad behavior.

I think that this may be a case of getting stuck in the lesson. The older I get the more things have stayed the same; my "getting into trouble" should have ended long ago. I was fed up. I decided that people could try, but it was up to me to not **feel** naughty anymore. That was the "Ah-hah!" I had to quit allowing myself to feel that I was in the wrong. It wasn't about the other person and what tone they used. It wasn't about getting the other person to change their behavior. It wasn't about making the other person happy ... or making them angry. If I could feel naughty in a room by myself, just because I dripped something on the floor, changing that was my job.

I'm not talking about extremes, but the issues of our daily ritual: the boss being a jerk; competition between peers; rallying people to take sides in a dispute; not meeting daily goals; coping with other people who are stressed out, while trying to handle our own stress.

Perhaps proper leadership skills aren't being taught; too many people think getting mad works. Some may believe that this is how it's supposed to be ... that being fierce, protective, and vigilant by requiring people to follow the rules fulfills the role of being an adult or a leader. Also, the belief that leadership's role is incentivizing other people, may be conducive to a better attitude, is still a control issue.

At any rate, I made a personal declaration, "I am not responsible for anyone's emotions." This may seem wrong in the midst of "stop the bullying" campaigns, but bear with me here. The point is that each of us is in charge of our own emotions.

No, I am not taking — nor granting — license to hurt people. Instead, I take my focus off people and place it on things. If people don't understand me and still want to act as if I offended them, then that is their problem. This goes hand in hand with knowing where my control really lies. I control myself and not them.

Now, I have to do my job, be honest, and stay in line. If I'm going to fight, I need solid ground to stand on so other people's control issues, tantrums, or attempts to bully do not affect me. No matter if it's offense or defense, it's the same formula. Use few words, be specific, and control things not people. It isn't a competition to see who can hurl the most slurs or trade the most barbs. Get to the point. Stay on topic. Be open to admitting that I can stand corrected. Anything else is ammunition that will be volleyed back and forth until we are both just angry. Basically, when someone goes on a tirade, I pretend they're communicating correctly and I take my focus off them and put it on what needs to be done. If they flew off the handle, and I easily complied —because that's what I'm supposed to be doing anyway — they look foolish for over-reacting.

Treating people as if they're naughty stands in the way of the real solution. One of my employers had an Employee Of the Month (EOM) program for day crew and another for night crew; the kicker was that in most of the stores, day crew had only four to six people on the roster and about fifteen on the night crew. With a high turnover in new employees, everyone could be EOM two or three times a year. We often teased each other about how it was their "turn" to get it.

Well, as teasing does, it got old. In one of the stores, the manager in charge of the EOM program quit choosing people. Then she bragged that she could yank the program because she was in control. After a few months, having proved her point, she resumed the program, again asserting her control by allowing us to have our privileges. Time had passed and people started teasing **her** about the rotation. I don't know why, because she had proved she had all the control, so we let her have another go at it. So she pulled the program all together. She had all the power, but no one cared about the program anymore.

If she hadn't been so self-involved with deciding the chosen one, and so eager to punish the "naughty" ones, she could have come up with a better way of choosing the EOM. She could have elected team members to celebrate their birthday, and another to mark the anniversary of their employment. That would've been a start to reinvigorate the EOM program. She could have come up with anything. Instead she chose to be difficult, because she felt it was more powerful.

From this Goodness exercise, I learned that if people judge me, and are unable to conduct themselves without getting upset, defensive, offensive, sour, mad, taking a stand, etc., that's their issue, not mine. I'm not that rotten of a person, so if that is their preferred relationship with me, that's their problem. I can't change it until they allow it to change. From now on I declare, I'm not naughty, naughty, naughty! I am an adult! I make decisions! If it's a bad decision? That's all it is, **a decision**!

I'm Not Naughty, Naughty, Naughty

As an adult I've stood against others who used their temper trying to get me to conform to rules that other **adults** developed. Now, since I am mindful that I'm "not naughty, naughty, naughty; I am an adult!" I have to go about my day, mindful that others aren't naughty, naughty, naughty, either. The part that's hard to remember is: what I give out might not be returned. But, now I have more good days than bad.

Goodness

Chapter 5   Recalibrate Your Definition Of A Good Day

From time to time I would think about the past and the present. I would think about how people used to go for Sunday drives and now we have road rage ... how people in the past are presented as happy but then got angry, and today, everybody is angry but looking to get happy. I found it futile to keep trying to have a good day ... day after day, after day, because other people and things would just come along and wreck it. In turn, this would make me angry, worried, or function on fear.

So what is your definition of a good day? Is it for everything to go click, click, click like clockwork with nothing to throw it off track? Are you living for occasions when your kids are well-behaved all day? No problems to encroach on your efficiency? No interruptions to your schedule and everything gets done on time? A day when traffic flows well, with no road rage and no trains holding you up at the crossing to make you late? All of this on the same day when you function efficiently; when you get up on time; go to bed on time; you cook and eat all three meals; provide healthy snacks; exercise; do your household chores; on the same day all bills are up to date; with time, money, and energy to spare for shopping and some family activities to boot?

Are you going along, living your good day, then — wouldn't you know it? — someone comes out of the blue who's decided you can't get by with that, then works very hard to extend their bad day onto yours? Does your day get bad because others don't know how to do their job, and in turn affect yours?

I wasn't looking for perfection ... I know some days are bad days just because they are bad. Besides, if there were no bad days, I wouldn't know what a good day looked like. But, if I am holding out for others to NOT make it a bad day, then I might be waiting for only a few good days a year.

I discovered that, if it's your problem, it's your problem; if it's my problem, then it's mine. It gets confusing when your problems are disguised as my problems. Some people are really good at that. This is where my focus on controlling **things** and not people is put to the test ... And it works.

For example, it seems as though people have forgotten how to ask for anything. I am not someone's minion, but I do know how to take direction if people need to ask something of me. Since I know how to take direction, other people should find it easy to ask, but instead, they will yell, dictate, command, or become passive-aggressive.

The catch is, I have to be honest: I may not always be presenting myself as one who easily takes direction. If someone asks me to do something and my response is, "Yeah I know," that kind of shuts them down. Sometimes, I think I say something in support but I'm just stating the obvious and it sounds like I'm balking at the request. If someone needs to coach me because I made a mistake, or because they felt I needed direction, instead of just letting them, I have caught myself making excuses, or trying to explain away my ditziness. I have also been on the other side where all I am trying to do is say what I need to say. In return, the other person is adding all this other stuff to the conversation and basically wasting time by extending the conversation.

What I find funny, is that I thought that I was protecting myself, or my intelligence, but in reality, if I got defensive, or grumbled that I was told, I had demonstrated that I wasn't able to take direction. I had merely fed their idea that they can't ask. I found it important to quit grumbling when I was "told" and to just shut up, and recognize that I am a good person. So I have to be honest that this **is** my problem.

Now, if I am not doing any of these things and they still yell, dictate, command, or become passive-aggressive, then that is their problem. There is nothing I can do about it, because it's their personal struggle with asking a question … asking for help, etc. Some people might be in the position where they feel they can't afford to "not know." This is their problem. They can yell all they want but I'm not going to act like I'm naughty, naughty, naughty. This takes practice and works when I am honest that it is **not** my problem.

This is a little like choosing your battles, but I don't want to say that, for fear people will start choosing **to** battle. Just wait to see **if** you really need to battle, because sometimes you do need to battle to defend yourself.

Goodness

This is the adage about holding a mirror to yourself. If you are bothered by every "eh" and "tsk" in a conversation, quit saying, "eh" and "tsk" to other people. If you are tired of being interrupted, quit interrupting. These old adages about battles and mirrors are there for a reason, so don't feel shame if you need to make a correction. Instead get curious, feel good. You are making changes to protect your good day.

There will be bad days that happen beyond your control, so the less you have a hand in creating them, the better. You can't protect your good day if you go around feeling naughty. This only works if you are coming from a place of "Goodness." This only works if you are honest.

Chapter 6   Honesty

None of these fruity experiments work to their full potential without honesty. There were times when I thought I had learned my lesson, then another lesson would reveal itself and I just kept finding more layers. There were times I felt I was doing the opposite of what I've learned growing up. During these times, honesty kept me grounded. Frankly, switching from hyper-vigilance and intense concern, to a perspective of calm and patience, felt like I had lost my sense of urgency. The people in my life thought I had, too.

I can point out a layer right there. While it shouldn't matter what people think, your spouse will notice a change. If they think that you've quit caring, because you quit worrying about everything, they will react accordingly. It might be important if your boss thinks you've lost a sense of urgency, even though you know you've become more efficient. When people second guess me and apply pressure to keep me doing the familiar, being honest with myself helps when I do care what people think.

Another layer revealed itself. Vigilance and constant concern are grounded in worry. I thought I was being pro-active. I thought I was being intelligent. I thought I had foresight. My goal was to never be caught off guard. I was always vigilant to ensure that it never happened again, whatever **"it"** was at any given moment. Letting all the worry go seemed as if I would be unprepared for any repercussions. It took a while to get over the feeling that I was being careless.

Being vigilant, concerned, pro-active and intelligent had been my rules to live by. This fruity project was becoming uncomfortable, as if I had dropped the ball and was dead weight for those around me. I felt like I was reversing the comfort of playing fair; I felt dishonorable when I stopped being accountable for everything, and I felt like I was ignoring the service of sacrifice. As these "ill" feelings tried to interrupt my work, honesty would keep me on track. I kept asking myself, "What is really going on here? What would happen if I dropped this ball just once? What would happen if I took one day to see what would happen if I weren't worried, if I weren't accountable? It's just one day and one event out of my entire life."

I got my answers. I made adjustments, such as, I'm not dead weight if I am doing my part and taking care of my own. When it comes to sacrifice, I can't give what I don't have, i.e., deficient is deficient. Trying to keep things fair just leads to controlling people and getting mad at them for being unfair and trying to force rules of fairness on them. Living life as unfair doesn't mean it's wrong; I merely gave up my role as judge about what is fair. For example, if I covered someone's shift so they could have the night off? The grateful response could be "I owe you one." Well, what if they didn't owe me one? What if I stepped out of the way and let things naturally fall into place?

Honesty

A really big layer was recognizing that lying **is** fear. You can argue with me all you want and say it is protection, especially via little white lies, or "it's nobody's business," but so far I haven't come across one case where lying doesn't originate in fear. The urge to lie is based in fear of consequences.

To protect — the word itself is to ward off the fear of harm and suffering. I think when it comes to lying we get that mixed up. We start thinking that the urge to lie is to **protect** from knowing the truth so it feels safe. We view being honest as getting into trouble, as in, "Yes, I did that naughty thing. Now I must be noble and tell the truth to serve my penance." It took some work to unravel that misnomer. Lying is not protecting. Being honest is not getting into trouble.

Believe me, I'm not striving to be goody-two-shoes, nor am I a perfectionist. I didn't work on honesty because I was a habitual liar. I thought I **was** honest. As it turned out, I pretty much lied all day. I lied to block that person, prevent this confrontation, be competitive, hide my B side, be full of energy when I was tired, and be worried when I didn't need to be. I was flooded with anxiety and I always wanted something else. I liked who I was, but I wanted to make changes to make me better.

Another layer I see daily, is that after doing all this work, I still lie. In fact, lying by omission has probably increased. I've heard that lying creates distance. Maybe in some circumstances I **want** that distance.

Since I am on the topic of lying on purpose, I quit "faking it until I make it." I found it to be a form of

dishonesty with myself. I suppose the words "faking it"
tipped me off. Now that I've noticed, I was able to track
what I really do. Let's say we have a simple face-to-face
conversation, but I'm moody. If I fake a smile, I feel false; I
feel like crap, I get stuck in that smile. You may sense it,
and return the fake exchange. Maybe something genuine
comes out of it, but still, I'm getting there via being mired in
crap.

What happens when I'm honest? Well, now that I have
an interest in protecting my good day, I want to leave the
bad mood and move on to the good mood. Also, I'm no
longer eager to wreck your day by infecting you with my
bad mood. I may not be smiling when I start this face to
face conversation, but as I am looking at you, I think of
how I want to present myself. This gets me out of my
head and puts me in the moment. My bad mood is moving
into the past and I'm in a new moment; a new mood
emerges. It depends on what transpires between us. In
short, I set a goal, then I act to meet that goal.

Of course, this is easier said than done. This is the
outline of what happens, not the actual action. From what
I have felt, there is no "faking it." In varying degrees, this
has helped when I need to be a good sport, when I'm
freaked out about trying something new, or in a scramble
and things aren't going as planned. I remind myself to
protect my good day and set a goal to get back into that
good spot.

This next layer changed my perspective. I was
watching a health show and the topic was cheating on
your diet. The segment showed women sitting in their car
revealing their stashes of candy that they ate when they

were alone, specifically, away from their husbands and children. They explained they wanted to lose weight and knew they should eat healthy, so now they feel naughty and guilty.

My change in perspective came when watching these videos: all I saw were women who were sitting in their cars alone, who had made the decision to buy a candy bar and eat it. These are adult women, grown ups. I get that this is a real problem ... and this problem is making them nervous, upset, doubtful. There's also probably some guilt going on that they had decided not to share with their kids, but still, **all I see is a woman who made a choice to eat the candy bar she bought**.

Quit celebrating naughty. You're an adult. You don't need to answer to anyone. You make choices. Eat the candy bar, add the calories in, and go on with your day. Naughty has nothing to do with it. For this reason I quit announcing to people that I am going on a diet, losing weight, exercising more, quitting smoking, writing a book, etc. Be honest and quit staging a role reversal to which you, **the adult,** are held accountable by your children for being naughty when you're caught "cheating." NO! The moms are the adults! Also, women say, "I don't have to answer to any man," then hold themselves accountable to their husbands because they made the choice to eat a candy bar?! What is that? So you answer to a man but only when it suits you? Think about it.

These are starting points, and not solutions. I first learned how to get comfortable with, "I'm not naughty, naughty, naughty." Then I saw what happened while being honest about it. I didn't say anything, nor tell anyone, nor come clean about my observations. I was only honest with myself while I pondered, thought, meditated, prayed, whatever I did, to think through what I really was doing.

My current experience is you should always, ALWAYS, **ALWAYS**, be honest with yourself. I'm not sure if you should always be bald-faced honest with other people, but I think you need to be honest with yourself about why you would lie ... And, I think I need to tell you, it doesn't hurt to know why. Remember, you made a decision to lie; it is not naughty, naughty, naughty. (If you go out and rob a bank, you're naughty ... If you lie to say you didn't do it, you're naughty ... duh.) But, if you don't like your friend's haircut and you're asked, "Do you like my hair?" then respond "Yes." Are you lying, out of fear of their reaction? Or because nothing can be done except wait for it to grow out? If you don't know, you don't know, but you should always ask yourself, why do I feel this need to lie and what would happen if I were honest? In fact when you get into facing the fear or asking why you have the urge to lie, or the urge to hide behind lying, this can lead to some pretty fascinating results. Don't fear. Get curious.

Conclusion

I hope you have noticed that this book hasn't been about Good and Evil. Evil is evil, breaking the law is breaking the law, hurting someone is hurting someone. These are not right.

Nor has this been about doing something naughty, then shouting out gleefully that you aren't naughty, as some people like to spin it. You can't be speeding down the road doing 55 mph in a 35 mph zone and start singing, "I'm an adult! I'm not naughty, naughty, naughty! I can do whatever I want. Woo-hoo!"

When you are constantly challenged with wrong, wrong, wrong, the saying, "I'm not naughty, naughty, naughty," is a defense to quit putting yourself in the position of feeling like a child when accused or challenged. If you want to protect your good day, you can't be running around feeling like you're naughty all the time. Take a day or two to get out of that childish mode. Practice once or twice not taking one for the team. Instead of feeling naughty because you did the wrong thing, treat it like a decision, and see how that feels. Does it open up options for other decisions you could make?

Goodness

I know I keep saying the same thing, but again, we forget that these aren't laws of nature. **We** humans put the rules in place so we can re-create that environment over and over again. Sometimes there are two or even three ways to do things, and all of them are "right" ways. When that happens, don't compete for which "right way" is "righter." These aren't lines drawn in the sand to determine who is good or bad. At the end of the day, we're just humans trying to get things done.

These discussions border on the topic of worthiness. When someone tells you that you are worthy, you know it's true. Of course you know you're worthy; you can feel it in your gut. It's like "duh."

But when we are bouncing from moment to moment, our worthiness gets drowned out in the present. We feel bad and wonder what went wrong, then we have a couple of normal moments, then the next moment have feelings of unworthiness, and the struggle continues. Those moments happen when we recognize that we didn't have fun today, or the paycheck wasn't enough, then more needs arise. It could be that our schedule is out of sync with the rest of the world, so we feel alone, and the needs of community and companionship go unmet. These are the moments we need to capture and say, "Wait a minute … I'm good, I'm here, so how do I proceed?"

Epilogue

I worked for a guy who would randomly call a quiet day. There were also days that weren't so random, such as when he had a clue that bad attitudes were lurking and the crap was about to hit the fan. To keep everyone on board with the idea, he would give happy reminders throughout his shift as if he were exclaiming that it was Friday, or something. "Yay, it's a quiet day. Today is going to be a good day."

Eventually "quiet days" easily became the norm. We had a good working experience during his shift and nobody really understood why. So when he left for the day and someone else took over, things weren't so great.

Here is my take. When he instilled quiet days, he was in charge of the environment. He wasn't babysitting a bunch of adults telling them to suck it up and get over it. He didn't tell people to quit whining ... grow up ... get a thicker skin ... or, do something about it. Instead, since employees had to be quiet, we had to rely on our own self-control to not latch on to the slightest "oops" about which to vent, rant, and complain. We just fixed it and moved on to a new situation that wasn't infected by the past situation. We weren't suppressing our feelings. Without latching onto negativity, there was nothing to suppress. Quiet days also worked for the opposite attitude. You couldn't be overly exuberant and screw around. We were there to work.

This manager set the standard for the environment and those who chose not to honor that standard met the consequences, which was outlined in our employee handbook -- you can look up whatever you agreed to in your own employee handbook.

During these "quiet days," the real choice for personal conduct was up to the employees. They chose to quit making mountains out of mole hills. If there was a problem, it was quietly fixed and everybody moved on. If it wasn't their problem, they stayed out of it and waited to be asked for help. If someone had a problem, they could stand up for themselves by calling a meeting away from the work area, in the office or the back room, and have a reasonable conversation without disrupting the quiet day. No showy displays of disgust were allowed. He set the standard. We chose to meet it. We **wanted** to protect our good day at work.

Bad work environments exist because people don't know how to train other adults to quit being a victim of circumstance. **Or**, they feel they shouldn't have to train in this topic because these people are old enough to know better, or it was their parent's job to train them. Controlling the environment helps to deal with these peculiarities in different manners, without the manager taking on a parental role. If the employee ever unreasonably challenges the authority of a manager, they should be fired, but everyone makes it more complicated than that.

Epilogue

If the manager doesn't resort to using the tools laid out in the employee handbook, then the manager is dealing with their own personal control issues. And it usually involves controlling other humans.

The best I could do at work was to make changes in myself since that is what I control. I didn't wait for employers to implement change in others. In fact with this new mindset the manager's relationship with other employees was none of my business. Yet still, I had seen positive shifts in my work environment. Those difficult exchanges in human interactions still go on all around me — all the time. This I can't control.

I think if organizations could find a way to incorporate these fruity principles into the training modules, we would see more women executives and women with higher wages, as these are the tools of negotiation and leadership. When these tools of virtues are in place, worry, fear, anger, and rules of fairness are unnecessary, because there is security in having control over oneself, which is exactly what you want when others are so unpredictable and so uncontrollable. When you can comfortably control yourself, you start spreading goodness. At least you have the choice. It starts with me and you, going out and making the best of it, even when we stumble and are faced with our worst. At the end of the day, we are good people who are just trying to get things done.

Goodness

Acknowledgments

Of course I'd like to thank my family for putting up with me all these years. Thank God he gifted me with you. I'd like to think if I'd had all this stuff down earlier, there would have been at least one less freak-out and maybe I would only have taken up one job instead of two and only held two jobs when I had three.

I'd like to thank Amazon for creating this incredible opportunity. You have reignited the idea that anything is possible in such a tangible way. It is there for us to just reach out and touch it.

I'd like to thank my editor, Dar Streedbeck; I couldn't have made the big crossover to "published" without you. I'd also like to thank my writing group. Not only have you given my spinning wheels traction in edit after edit, but my subject matter stands up when I hold it against our group. When we meet, our writing transcends from being so secret, so personal, and so guarded to being exposed to other people. What's more, it is exposed in a place where the writing is to be scrutinized, ripped apart and threatened. This should be the place where all the bickering, hen pecking and wounded egos happen, but it's not. We explore the creativity of other people's opinions. We thank each other for the corrections so our piece doesn't go out into the greater public with all our flaws. We laugh through the entire meeting, we go home feeling inspired and we can't wait until we meet again.

Thank you.